Breast CANCER

AWARENESS BOOKLET

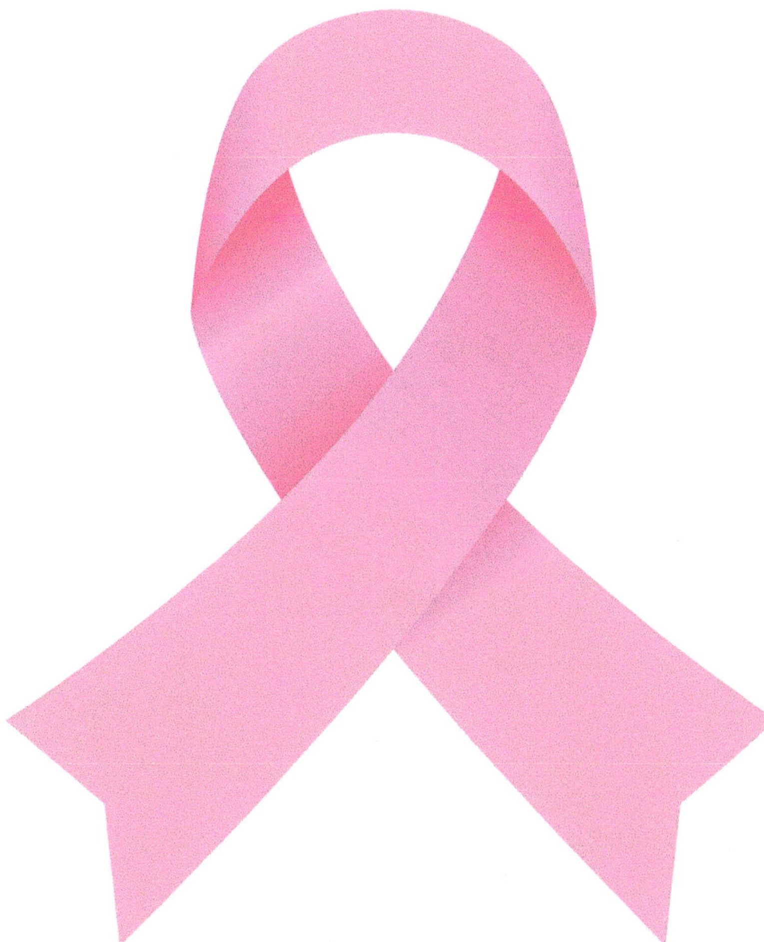

EMPOWERING THROUGH KNOWLEDGE AND SUPPORT

RAISING AWARENESS. SAVING LIVES.

Wear pink to support the fight against breast cancer.

WRITTEN BY DELATRIA SAM

ISBN: 979-8-3303-2046-2

To every warrior who has faced breast cancer with courage and grace—
This booklet is for you.
To the survivors whose scars speak of battles fought and won,
To those still in the fight, whose strength humbles and inspires,
To the loved ones who held vigil, whispered prayers, and wrapped hope around the hardest days,
To the souls we've lost, your light is eternal, your love still felt in quiet moments and laughter.
To all my loved ones I've lost to breast cancer, your memory is stitched into every page.
You are the reason I write, the reason I rise, the reason I believe healing is possible.
To the healthcare workers who show up with open hearts, who carry grief and grace in equal measure,
and offer care that goes beyond medicine,
thank you for being the quiet heroes in rooms filled with fear and hope.
May these pages be a balm.
May they remind us that we are never alone.
May they honor the truth: your story matters, your life matters, your love endures.
~Delatria Sam

Welcome Message

October is recognized as Breast Cancer Awareness Month, a time to raise visibility, share knowledge, and extend deep compassion to all those impacted. Whether you are walking through a diagnosis, supporting a loved one, grieving a loss, or simply seeking understanding, please know this: you are not alone.

This cancer awareness booklet was created with the intention of offering a compassionate and empowering resource for those impacted by breast cancer. It provides:

- *Personal stories that reflect courage, hope, and lived experiences*
- *Accessible information about breast cancer and its physical, emotional, and social impact*
- *Journaling prompts to encourage reflection. Coloring pages. Word games and brain teasers to keep your mind engaged and uplifted*
- *Resources for support, healing, and connection, designed to guide individuals, families, and caregivers through each stage of the journey.*
- *Visuals, survival stories, testimonials, tips, caregiver support info*
- *FAQs: Frequently Asked Questions about cancer, and more*
- *Nutrition and Wellness recommendations*
- *Patient Empowerment Message*
- *Dialogue: Conversation between a healthcare provider and her patient*
- *A Cancer Wish List: a heartfelt section where readers can write their wishes, hopes, or prayers*
- *Research Update, How to Get Involved Information*
- *Love Letter: Heartfelt letters from loved ones, a friend, and the person diagnosed with breast cancer.*
- *A Medical Glossary: Definitions of medical terms*
- *Memorial Page*

This booklet is more than a collection of facts; it's a space for reflection, encouragement, and community. Whether you're navigating a diagnosis, supporting a loved one, or honoring someone you've lost, these pages were made with you in mind.

With love and support,
Delatria Sam
Advocate, Loved One

STORY 1: SARAH'S JOURNEY

"When I was 35, my world shattered with the words 'you have breast cancer.'
I felt like I'd been punched in the gut, gasping for air.
This can't be happening to me, I'm too young, too healthy, too alive.
The diagnosis was a cruel wake-up call, forcing me to confront my own mortality.
But as I navigated the darkest days of treatment, I discovered an army of loved ones standing behind me, my family, who held my hand through every tear and every treatment; my friends, who showed up with food, prayers,

and listening ears; and my medical team, who fought alongside me with compassion and expertise. Their love and support were my lifeline, reminding me that I wasn't alone in this fight. Breast cancer may have taken parts of me, but it will never define me. Now, I'm driven to share my story, to spread awareness, and to urge others to get screened. If you're walking this path, know that you're seen, you're heard, and you're strong. Don't be afraid to lean on others – their love can be the very thing that carries you through."

STORY 2: MARK'S SUPPORT

“When my wife's doctor uttered those two words – 'breast cancer', my world crumbled. Overnight, our life together was turned upside down, and I felt helpless. As her caregiver, I wanted to be her rock, her safe haven, but I was lost. I didn't know how to support her, how to ease her pain, or how to be there for her in the ways she needed most.

Through the long, grueling days of treatment, I learned that sometimes it's the smallest acts of love that mean the most, holding her hand through chemo, listening to her fears and tears, being present in the darkness. It wasn't easy, but witnessing her strength, courage, and resilience inspired me to be stronger, to be better, and to be there for her when she needed me most.

Now, I want to urge others to stand by their loved ones as they go through this journey. Your support, whether it's driving them to appointments, cooking meals that bring them comfort, or simply being a shoulder to cry on, can be the difference between darkness and light. Breast cancer doesn't just affect the person diagnosed; it ripples through families, friendships, and lives. But with love, support, and awareness, we can face it together."

BREAST CANCER
What is it?

Breast cancer is a type of cancer that develops in the breast tissue when abnormal cells grow and multiply uncontrollably, forming a tumor. It can affect one or both breasts and can occur in both women and men, though it's more common in women.

BREAST CANCER

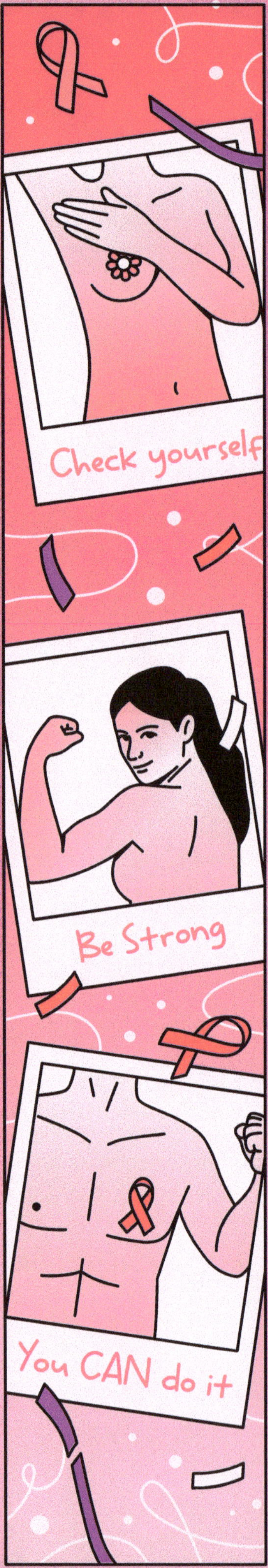

Join us to EMPOWER, EDUCATE, AND SUPPORT for

BREAST CANCER AWARENESS

BREAST CANCER FACTS:

- **STATISTICS: DID YOU KNOW THAT 1 IN 8 WOMEN WILL DEVELOP BREAST CANCER IN THEIR LIFETIME? ACCORDING TO THE AMERICAN CANCER SOCIETY, BREAST CANCER IS THE MOST COMMON CANCER AMONG WOMEN IN THE UNITED STATES.**
- **RISK FACTORS: RISK INCREASES WITH AGE, FAMILY HISTORY, GENETIC MUTATIONS, AND CERTAIN LIFESTYLE FACTORS.**

DETECTION METHODS:

- **MAMMOGRAMS: REGULAR SCREENING CAN HELP DETECT CANCER EARLY.**
- **SELF-EXAMS: KNOW YOUR BODY AND REPORT ANY CHANGES TO YOUR DOCTOR.**

TREATMENT OPTIONS: TREATMENT OFTEN INCLUDES SURGERY AND CHEMOTHERAPY. RADIATION, HORMONE THERAPY, OR TARGETED THERAPY, DEPENDING ON THE TYPE AND STAGE OF CANCER.

Let's focus on hope for early detection, better treatment, and a life without breast cancer. Show our unity and strength by lighting up our city in pink to spread awareness and support those affected.

APA Reference:

American Cancer Society. (n.d.). Retrieved from https://www.cancer.org

Q: What are some common symptoms of breast cancer?

A: Lump or thickening in the breast or underarm area, changes in the size or shape of the breast, nipple discharge or turning inward, skin changes like dimpling or redness.

TESTIMONIAL

"I was diagnosed with breast cancer at 35, and with treatment and support, I'm thriving today."

Kate Miller

TESTIMONIAL

“My mom’s breast cancer journey taught me the value of family support and staying positive.”

Lisa Jacobs

TESTIMONIAL

"During my treatment, I found that staying connected with loved ones and practicing self-care helped me cope with the emotional and physical challenges."

Kellie White

NOURISHING BODY AND MIND: SELF CARE

Prioritize Your Well Being with These Simple Steps

Find Peace During Treatment

Engaging calming activities like writing, meditation, or yoga, or talking to a friend, make time for activities that nourish your mind, body, and soul, which can help during breast cancer treatment.

Rest and Recover

Getting enough sleep is essential for mental and physical health to help manage fatigue during breast cancer treatment. Aim for 7-9 hours of sleep every night and create a relaxing bedtime routine to ensure quality sleep.

Prioritize Your Health

Learn to say no and set healthy boundaries for yourself. Maintain a balance between work, family, and time for yourself so you don't feel overwhelmed.

Nutrition & Wellness

Advice from a Registered Dietitian

“During treatment, I found that eating a balanced diet rich in fruits, vegetables, and whole grains helped me maintain my energy and overall health. Try to limit processed foods and added sugars.”

Sanctuary of Strength: A Warrior's Refuge

Think about a place where you felt completely safe and at peace during your journey with breast cancer. Describe this place in as much detail as you can. What did it look, sound, and smell like? How did you feel when you were there? Write down any memories or feelings that come to mind when you think about this safe space. How can you bring elements of this space into your current life and help you cope with challenges? You are a warrior, and your strength is rooted in your resilience, courage, and the love that surrounds you. Hold onto these feelings of safety and peace, and let them guide you through the ups and downs of your journey.

Pink Warrior Coloring

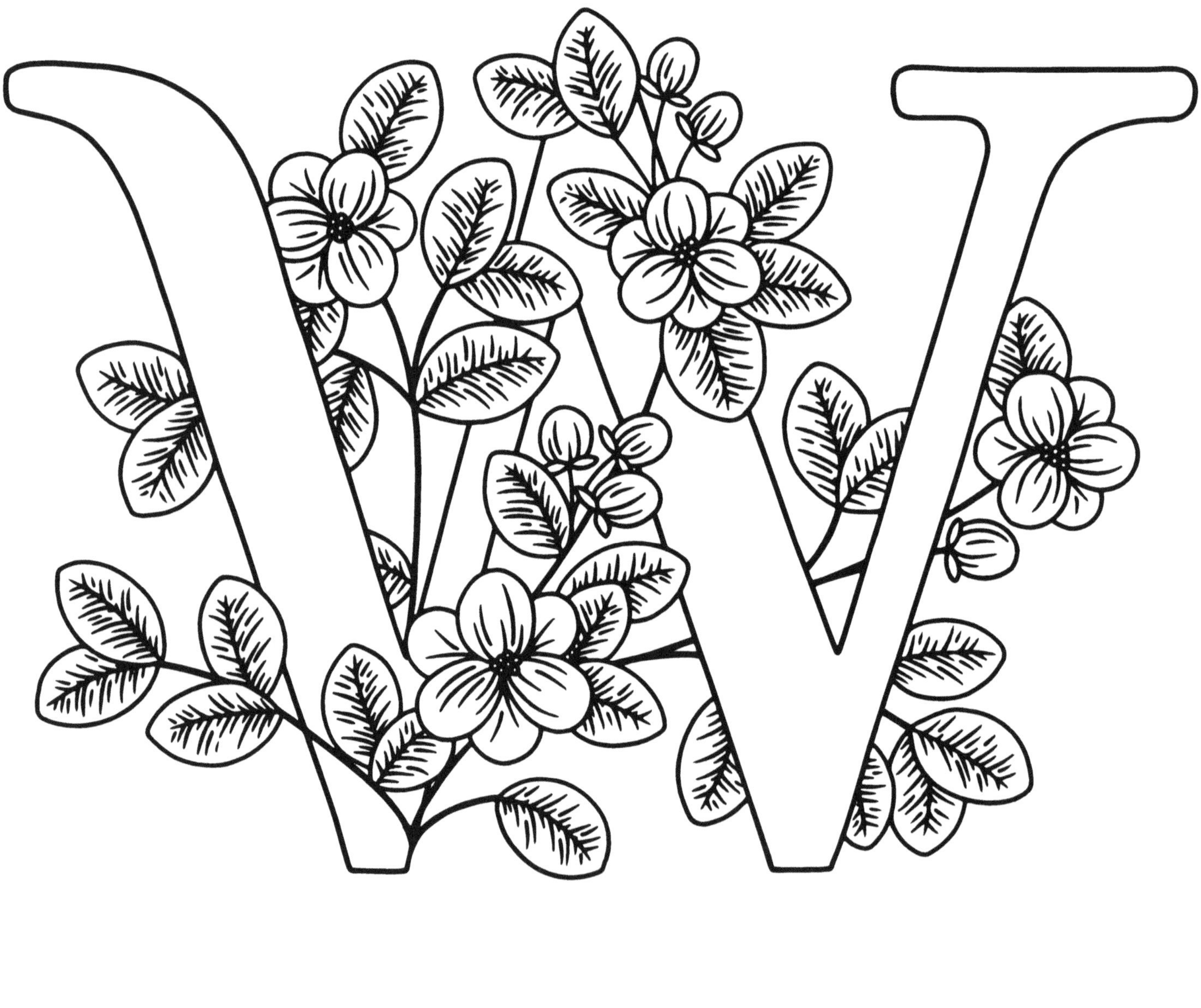

PATHWAYS TO HOPE

Find words symbolizing strength & hope in breast cancer.

Triumph
Support
Inspire
Stronger
Resilience
Warrior
Empower
Peace
Breast
Strength
Courageous
Caregiver
Care
Hope
Survivor
Victory
Love
Healing
Faithful
Remission
Cure
Brave
Determined
Cancer

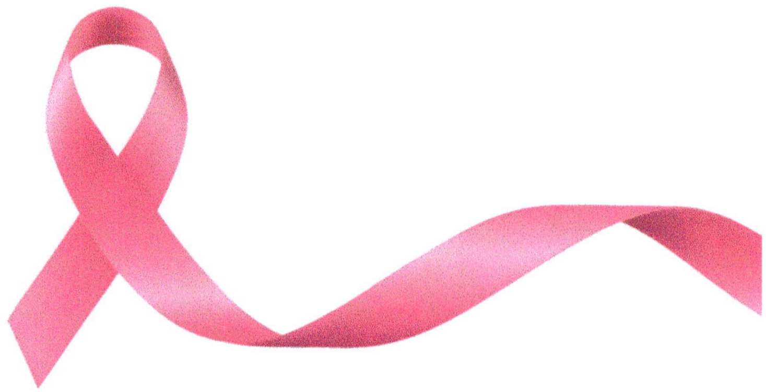

Breast Cancer Awareness:

PHYSICAL, EMOTIONAL, AND SOCIAL IMPACT

Physical Impact:
lump detection, nipple changes, hair loss, fatigue, pain, lack of energy, weakness

Social Impact:
relationship changes, treatment can impact work, social activities and daily routines. Importance of support groups, friends, and family

Emotional Impact:
fear, anxiety, trauma, overwhelmed, changes in self-esteem, changes in overall mood and behavior

Awareness & Support:
Resources: organizations, hotlines, and online communities.
Community involvement: fundraising, events, and awareness campaigns

Finding Strength in the Fight Against Breast Cancer

Think about a moment when you or someone you love showed incredible strength and courage in the face of breast cancer, whether it was during treatment, a doctor's appointment, or a tough conversation. How did that moment show your ability to endure and overcome challenges? Write about what you learned from that experience and how it continues to inspire you today.

Petal Path to Pink Strength Coloring

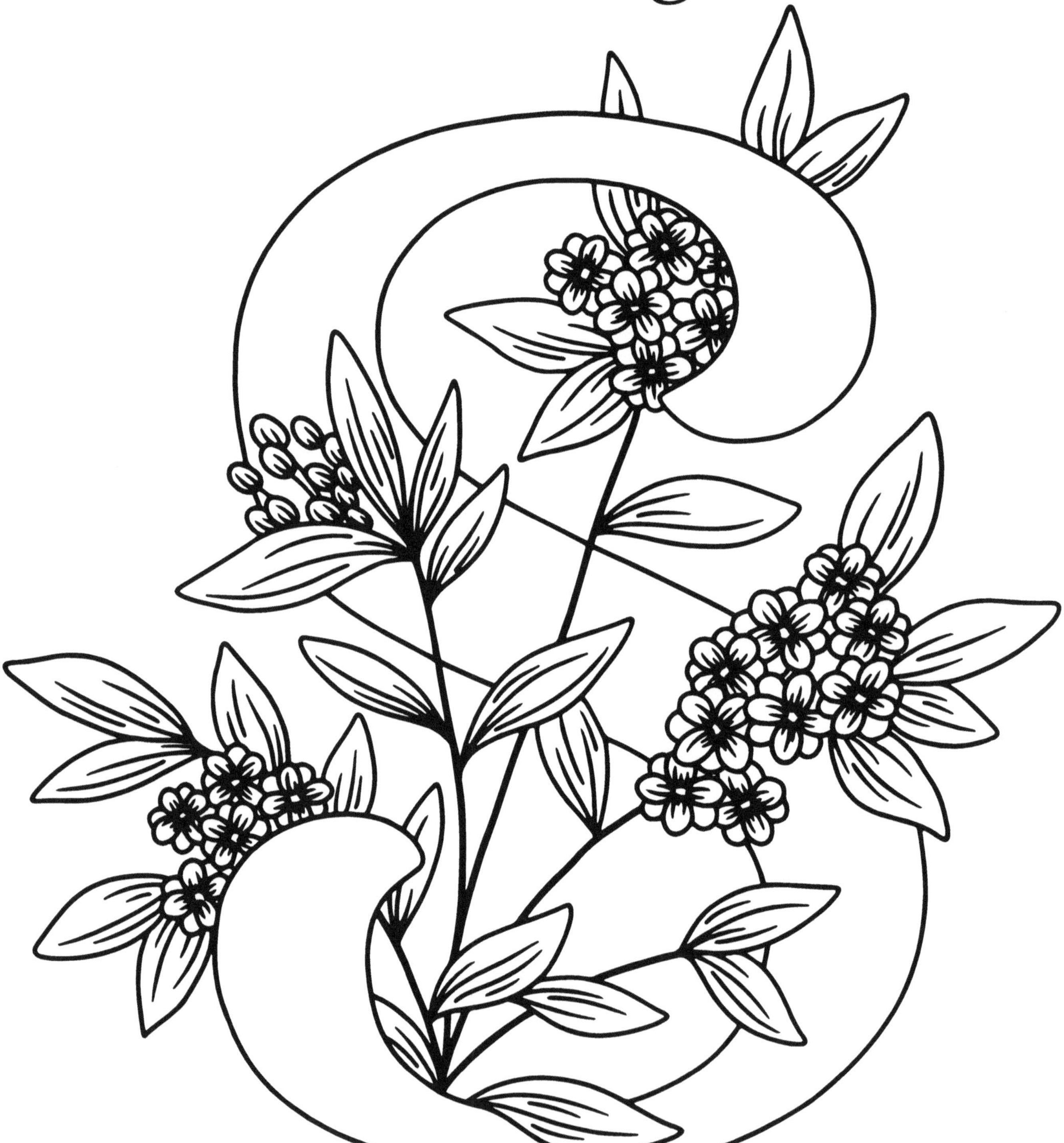

Q: Why is early detection of breast cancer important?

A: Because it increases the chances of successful treatment and survival. Regular screenings can help detect breast cancer at an early stage, often before symptoms appear. This allows for more effective treatment options and better outcomes.

STANDING STRONG TOGETHER AGAINST BREAST CANCER: SUPPORT, HOPE & HEALING

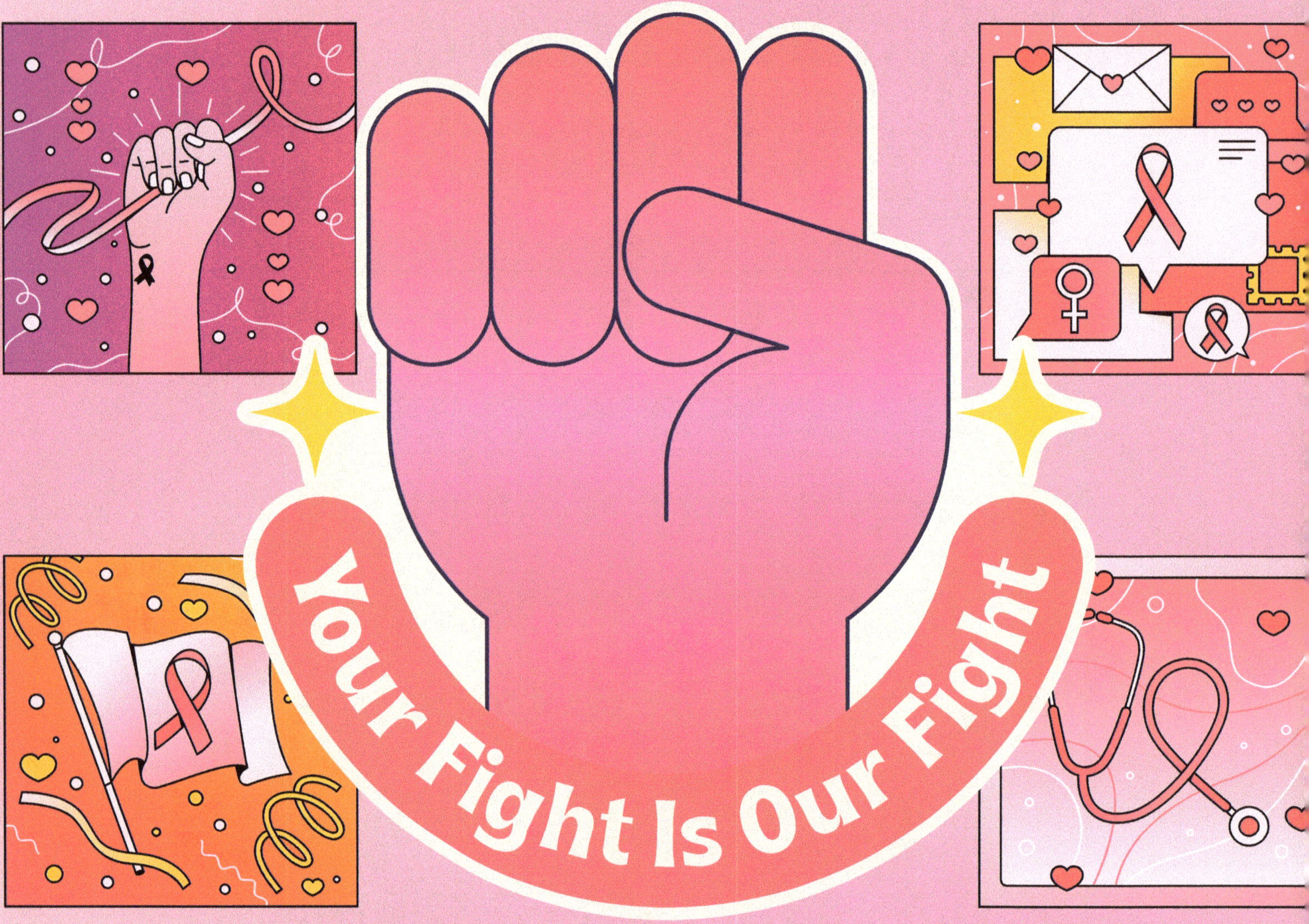

Breast cancer resources can provide vital support, healing, and connection for individuals, families, and caregivers navigating each stage of the journey.

BREAST CANCER SUPPORT RESOURCES

Social Connections:

Breast Cancer Survivor Socials: In-person and virtual events where survivors can connect, share experiences, and find support.

Breast Cancer Champions Free Community Events: Community events focused on health, wellness, and connection for breast cancer patients, survivors, and caregivers.

Pink the Park: A community event or fundraiser that brings people together to support breast cancer awareness and research.

Health and Wellness:

Wellness for Life: Offers mobile health services, including mammogram screenings, to promote early detection and prevention.

Treatment and Research:

Breast Cancer Clinical Trials: Research studies that explore new treatments, medications, and therapies for breast cancer. Patients can discuss clinical trial options with their healthcare provider to learn more.

Summits and Conferences:

Survivorship Summits: Events designed to empower survivors with knowledge, resources, and support for life after breast cancer.

Financial Assistance:

Financial Assistance Programs: Some organizations offer financial aid to help with treatment costs, transportation, and other expenses related to breast cancer care.

Creative Expression and Healing:

Art and Painting: Creating art can be a therapeutic outlet for breast cancer patients and survivors, helping to express emotions, reduce stress, and promote healing. Many organizations offer art therapy programs specifically designed for those affected by breast cancer.

Sharing Experiences through Writing:

Becoming a Breast Cancer Staff Writer: Sharing personal experiences, insights, and information about breast cancer can be a powerful way to support others going through similar journeys. By becoming a staff writer, individuals can:

Raise Awareness: Educate others about breast cancer, its impact, and the importance of early detection and treatment.

Provide Support: Offer emotional support and practical advice to patients, survivors, and caregivers through written content.

Build Community: Connect with others who have experienced breast cancer, creating a sense of community and solidarity.

Empower Others: Inspire and empower individuals to take control of their health, navigate treatment options, and advocate for themselves and others.

The Power of Determination: Holding On When Everything Feels Fragile. Determination is the heartbeat of survival, the quiet force that pushes us forward when fear, fatigue, and uncertainty threaten to pull us under.

Explore how determination shows up in the breast cancer journey, not just in treatment decisions, but in everyday moments: choosing to get out of bed, asking for help, advocating for care, or simply believing healing is possible. Reflect on how determination has shaped your own path or the path of someone you love. What does it look like when strength is quiet? When hope feels hard-won?

Determination in Pink: Finding Determination Through Breast Cancer Challenges Coloring

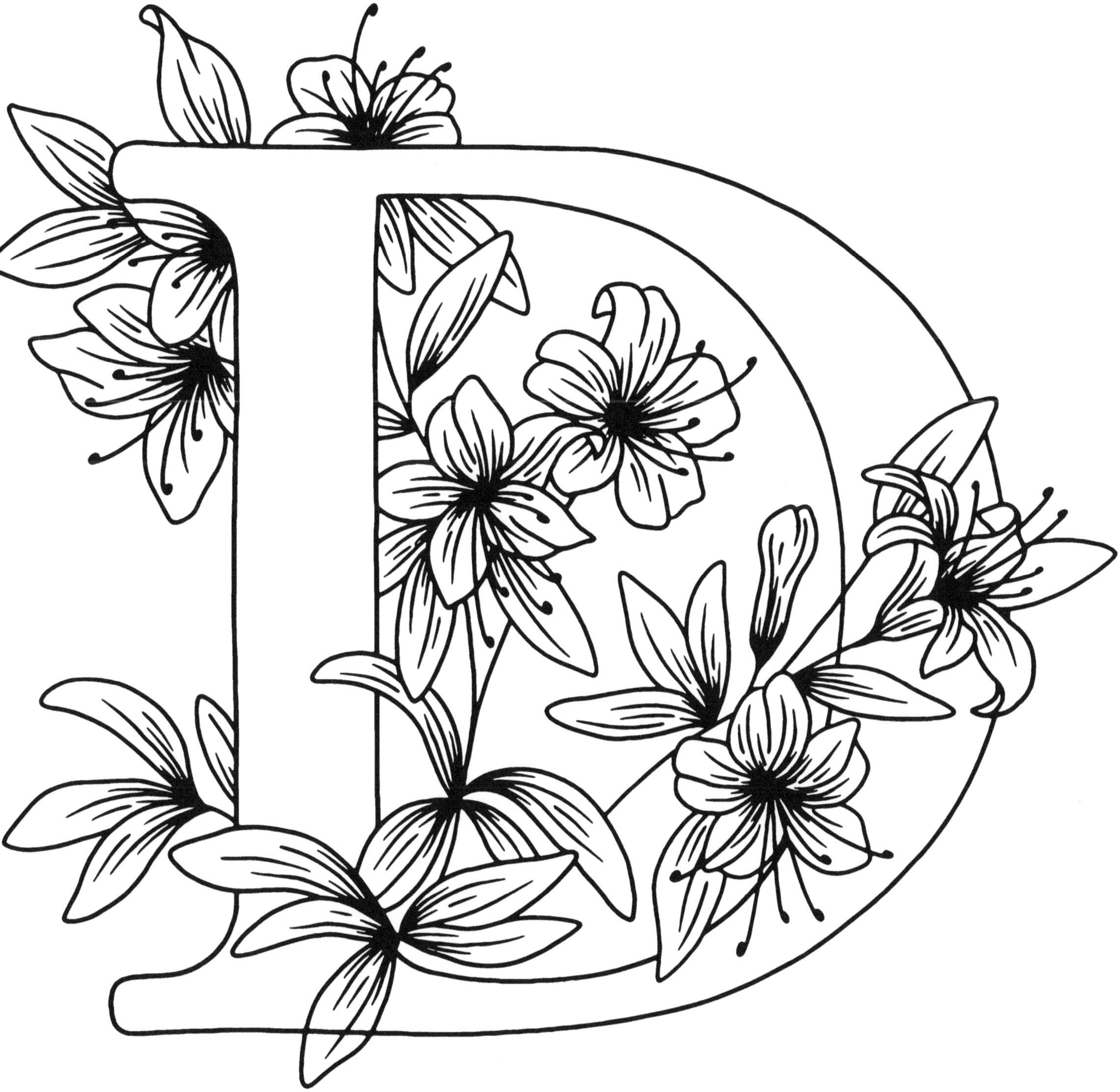

Courage in the Face of Challenge

Write about a moment when you felt courageous during your breast cancer journey. What did you do, and how did it make you feel? Reflect on how that courage has helped you navigate challenges and what it means to you moving forward.

Color Your Courage

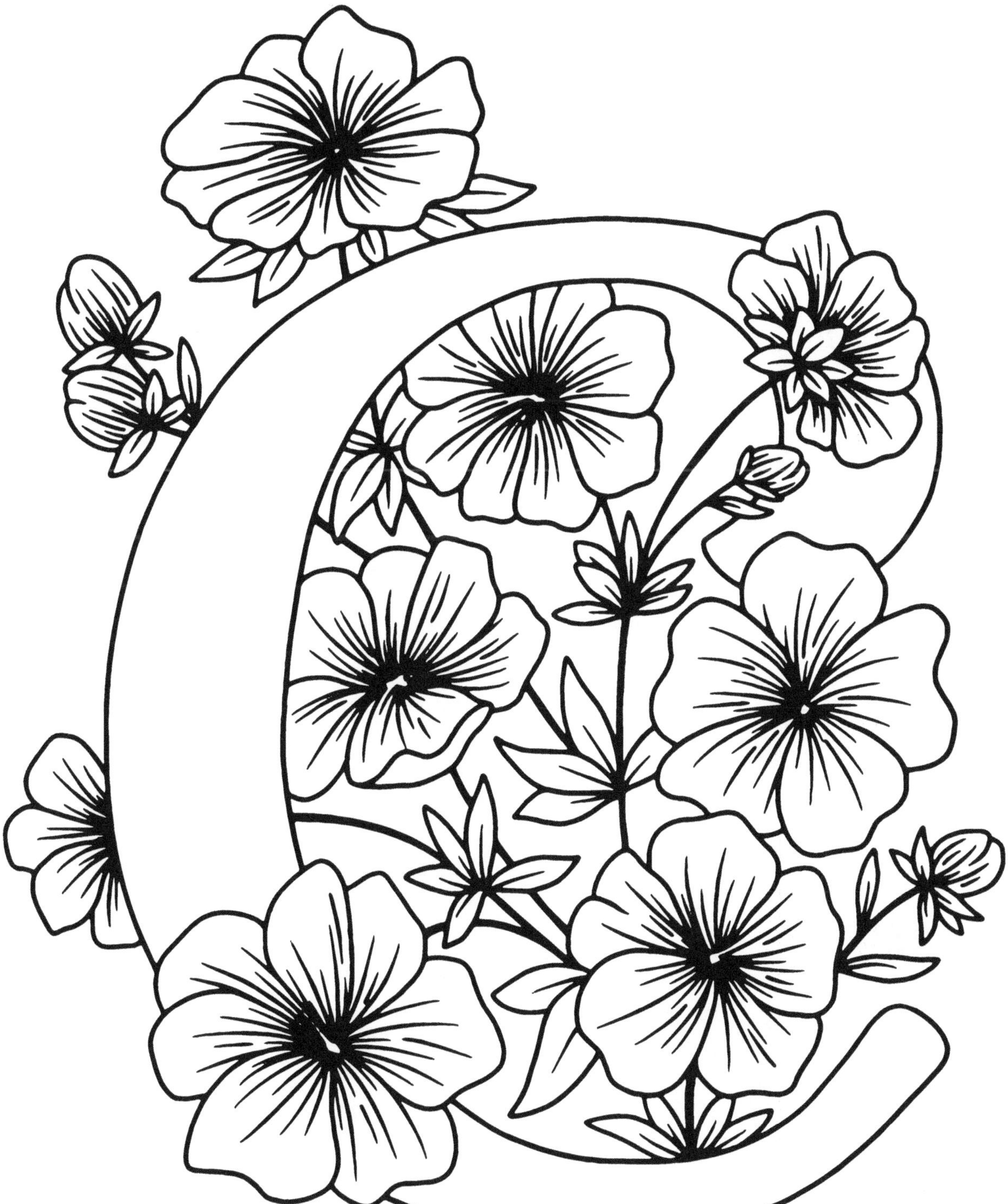

UNSCRAMBLE THE CURE

Set a timer for 5 minutes, and unscramble as many words as possible within the time limit.

MARGOMMAM ____________________

YPTHRAEMOEHC ____________________

YBIOPS ____________________

NOITADIAR ____________________

ITCNEEG ____________________

GTSAE ____________________

NCSAS ____________________

MOENRHO ____________________

URTOM ____________________

IECCEMAR ____________________

RRUCNCEEER ____________________

GGIMNIA STETS ____________________

Q: What are the benefits of genetic testing for breast cancer?

A: It can identify inherited mutations, such as BRCA1 and BRCA2, that increase the risk of breast cancer.

PREVENTION PALS CHECKUP

Have it checked

EARLY DETECTION SAVES LIVES.

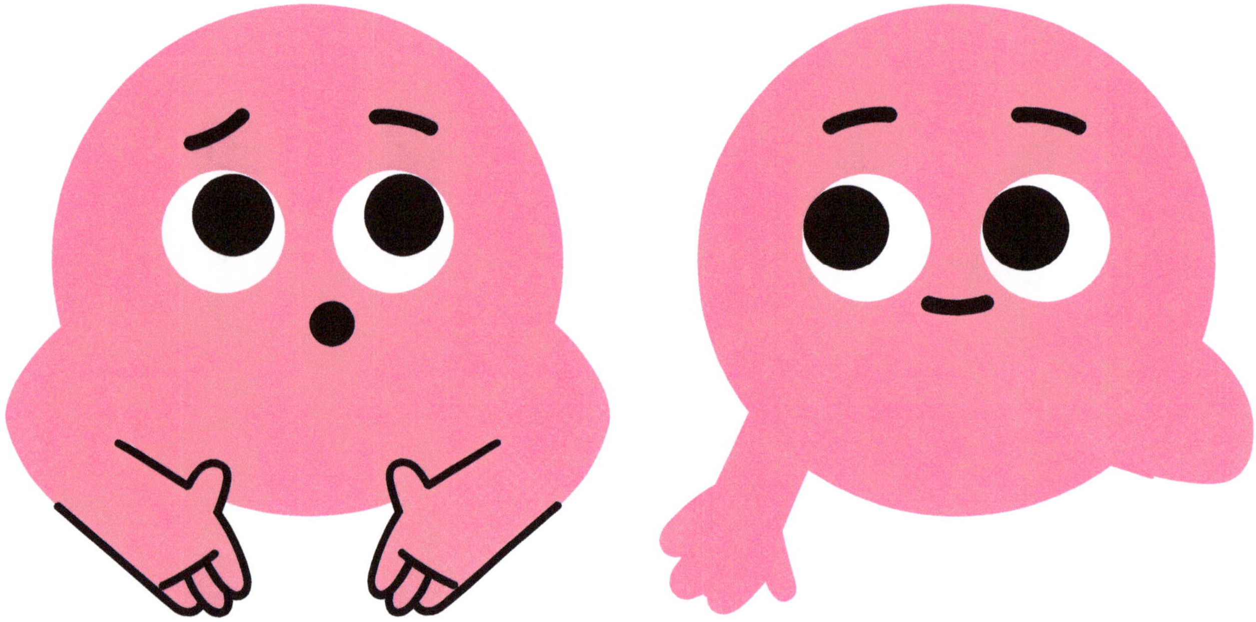

SCHEDULE YOUR MAMMOGRAM TODAY!
DO MONTHLY SELF-EXAMS.
KNOW YOUR FAMILY HISTORY.

Pink Ribbon Craft & Wear

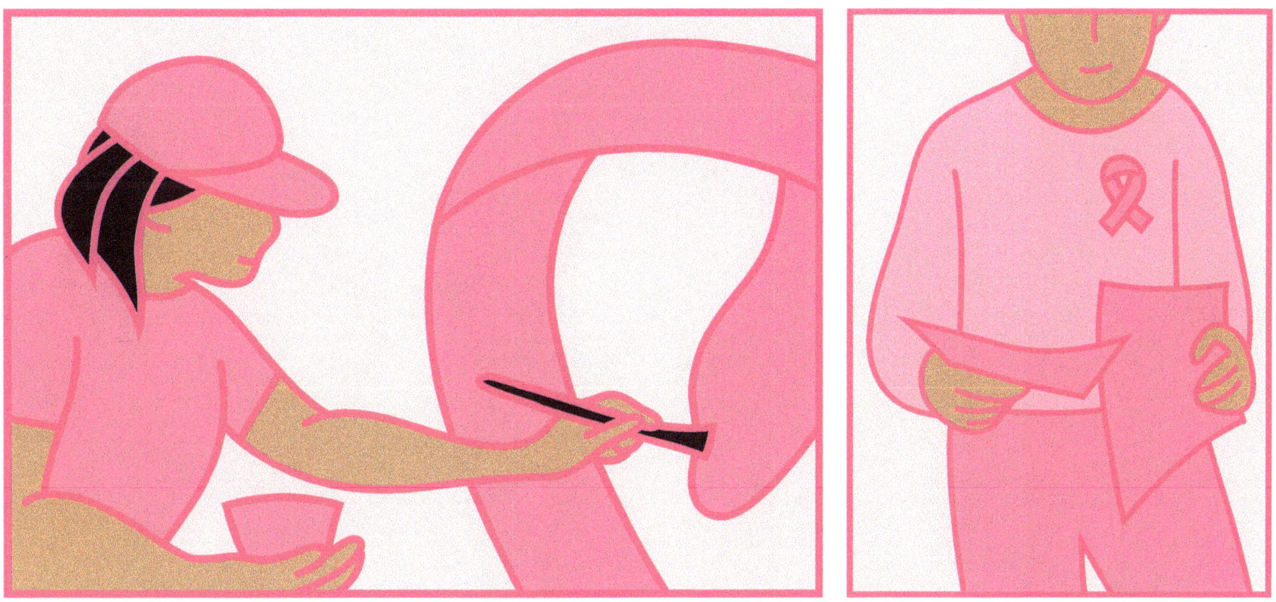

Encourage people to create their own pink ribbons. Then, have them wear the ribbons or pink outfits.

Pink Values Campaign

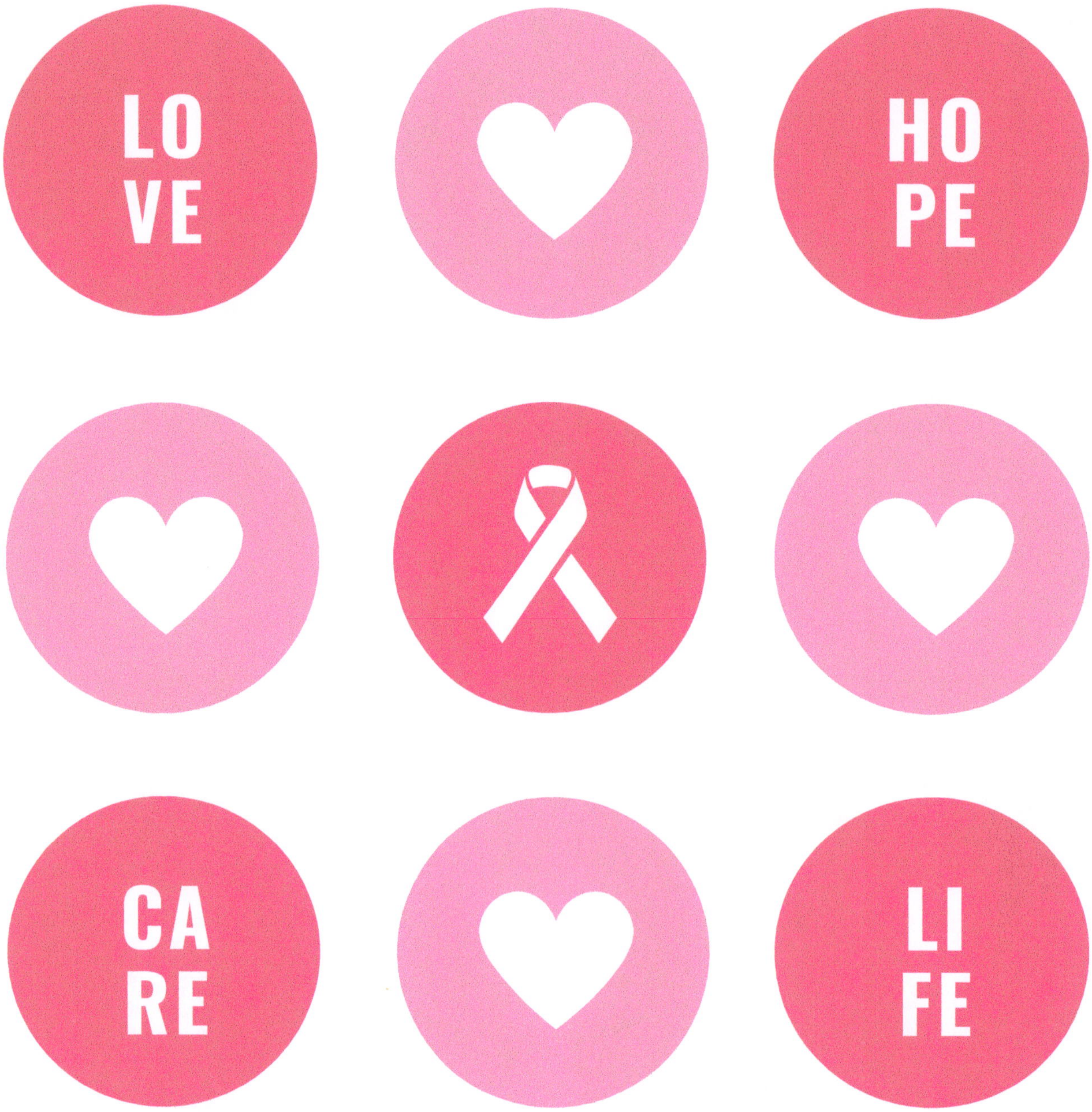

CHOOSE A VALUE: PICK ONE OF THE VALUES FROM THE PINK CIRCLES THAT RESONATES WITH YOU. DESIGN A PINK-THEMED POSTER OR SOCIAL MEDIA POST THAT HIGHLIGHTS YOUR CHOSEN VALUE.

Spread the word: Share your post using #PinkValues #BCAwareness and encourage others to join in.

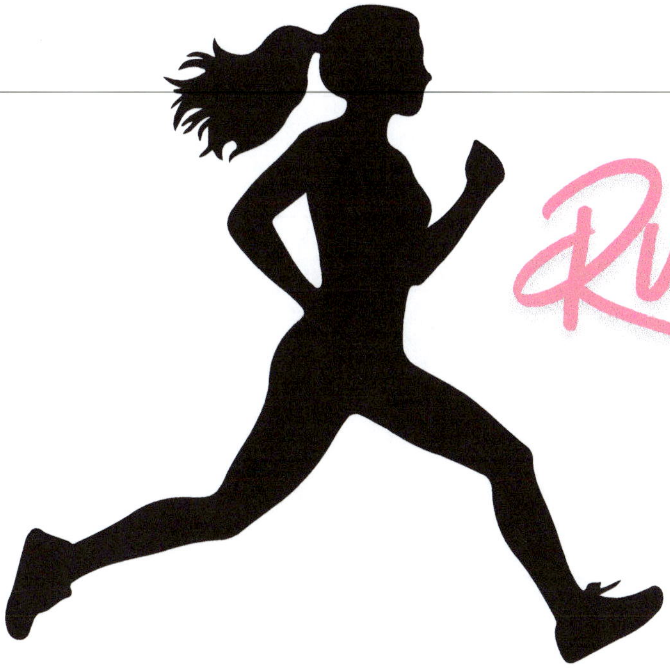

Run for the pink Ribbon!

Did you know running may lower the risk of breast cancer recurrence?

It improves survival rates, manages treatment side effects and enhances physical health.

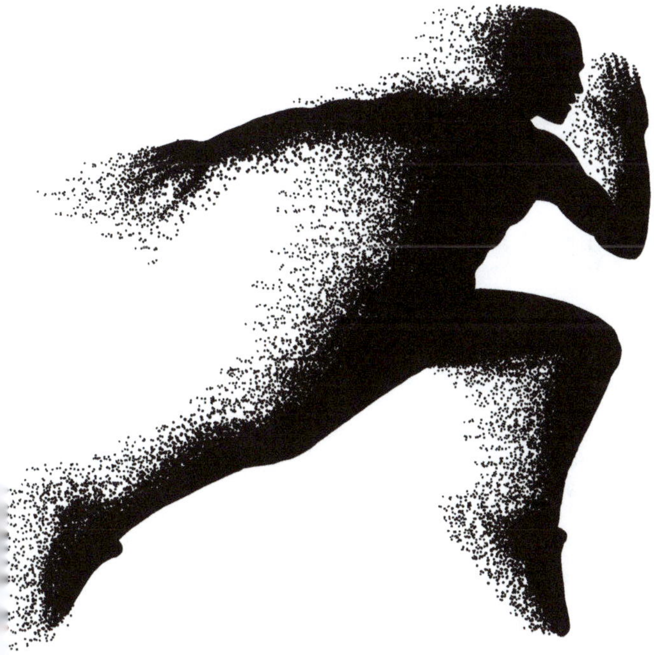

Consult healthcare providers before starting any new exercise program, especially during or after treatment.

RUNNING CAN BOOST MENTAL WELL-BEING

Q: What support options are available for breast cancer patients?

A: Survivorship programs, online resources and communities, counseling or therapy, in-person or virtual support groups, healthcare team (oncologists, nurses, nutritionists).

CREATE ILLUSTRATIONS OF PINK RIBBONS OR BRAS. SHARE YOUR ARTWORK ON SOCIAL MEDIA OR AT A LOCAL EVENT TO PROMOTE AND ENCOURAGE OTHERS TO GET SCREENED.

Feel Your Bumps For Lumps

Finding Comfort in Soothing Sounds

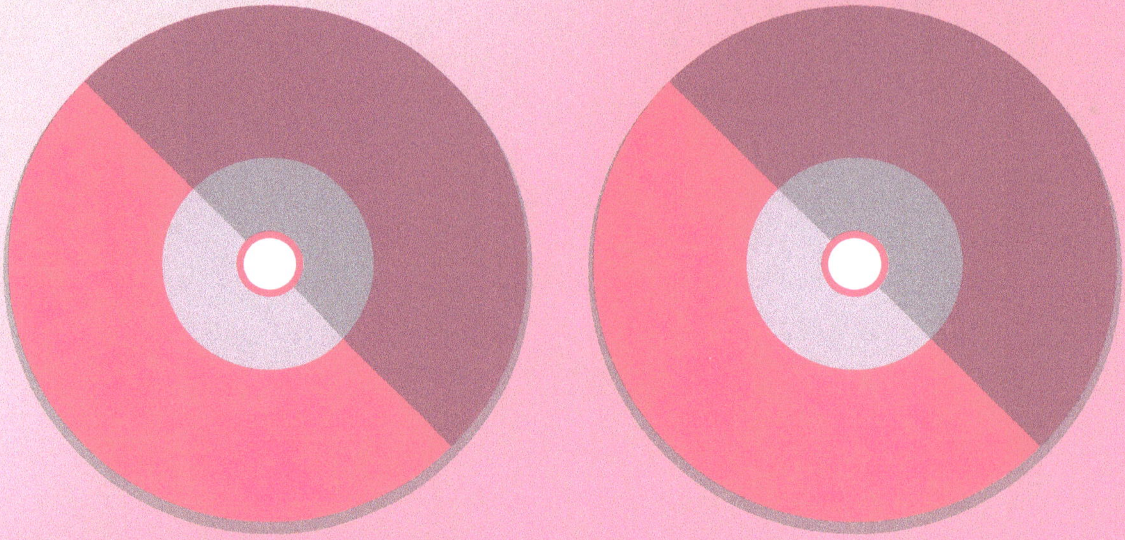

Listening to soothing music can be a powerful tool for those affected by breast cancer.

CREATE A PLAYLIST OF SOOTHING MUSIC. SHARE WITH OTHERS OR USE IT PERSONALLY FOR STRESS RELIEF.

HOPES FOR HEALING & SUPPORT IN THE FIGHT AGAINST BREAST CANCER.
WRITE DOWN HOPES OR WISHES NEXT TO THE NUMBERED HEARTS. CHECK THE BOXES AS YOU WORK TOWARDS OR RECEIVE SUPPORT.

1 ☐

2 ☐

3 ☐

4 ☐

5 ☐

6 ☐

7 ☐

8 ☐

9 ☐

10 ☐

BREAST TALKS: CONVERSATION BETWEEN THE HEALTHCARE PROVIDER AND THE PATIENT

HEALTHCARE PROVIDER	PATIENT
"Good morning, I'm Dr. Smith. How can I help you?"	"Hi, Doc. I've been having some concerns about breast cancer due to my family history."
"We'll do our best to help. As a patient here, you have certain rights & responsibilities. You have the right to be treated with dignity and respect."	"That sounds good. What are my options for breast cancer screening and diagnosis?"
"We offer mammograms, ultrasounds, and biopsies. We'll discuss the best approach for you based on your medical history and risk factors."	"Okay, got it. What about treatment options if I do have breast cancer?"
"We'll discuss surgery, chemotherapy, radiation, and other options. We'll work together to create a personalized treatment plan."	"Thanks for explaining everything, Doc. I feel more informed and supported."
"That's what we're here for. Let's take care of your health and get you the support you need."	"Ok, I'll make sure to schedule my mammogram soon based on what we discussed. Thanks again for your help."

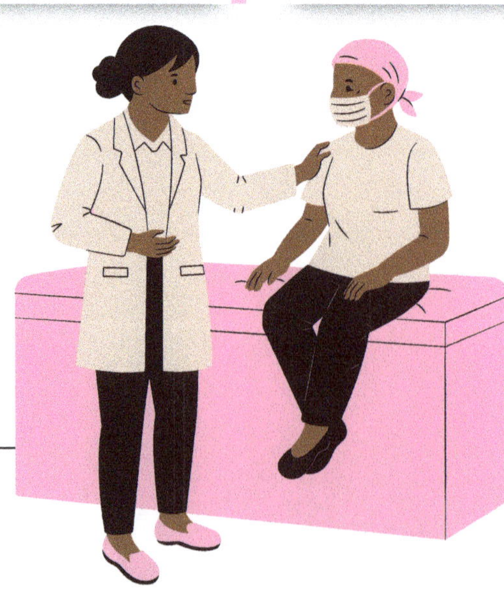

Q: What is the difference between invasive and non-invasive breast cancer?

A: Invasive breast cancer: cancer cells have spread into surrounding breast tissue & potentially to other parts of the body. Non-invasive cancer cells are confined to milk ducts or lobules and haven't spread to surrounding tissue.

RESEARCH UPDATE

Researchers are exploring new treatments for breast cancer, including targeted therapies and immunotherapies. Stay informed about the latest developments and discuss potential options with your healthcare team.

Breast Cancer

Love Letters

WRITING BREAST CANCER LOVE LETTERS CAN BE A THERAPEUTIC AND MEANINGFUL WAY TO EXPRESS EMOTIONS, PROVIDE COMFORT, CREATE A LEGACY, AND PROCESS EMOTIONS. THESE LETTERS CAN BE A POWERFUL WAY TO CONNECT WITH OTHERS, FOSTER EMPATHY, AND PROMOTE HEALING.

MY DEAREST

As you navigate this journey, I want you to know how much I admire your strength and resilience. I'm here for you, always. Your diagnosis doesn't change how much I love and cherish you; it only makes me more grateful for our time together.

I'm proud of you for facing this challenge head-on. Remember, you're not alone, I'm by your side every step of the way. I love you more than words can say.

YOURS ALWAYS

MY DEAR CHILD

as I go through treatment, I want you to know how much you mean to me. You're my inspiration. I'm fighting this cancer for us, for our future, and for the memories we'll create together.

Don't worry about me; I'll be okay. Focus on living your life to the fullest. I love you more than anything in this world.

WITH ALL MY LOVE, MOM

FROM A FRIEND

I'm sorry you're going through this, but I want you to know that you're not alone. I'm here for you, always. Whether it's a phone call, a visit, or just a listening ear, I'm here to support you.

You're strong, brave, and loved. Your diagnosis doesn't define you; your courage and resilience do. I'm honored to be your friend and to stand by you through this journey.

WITH LOVE AND SUPPORT

DEAR MOM,

As you face this challenge, I want you to know how much I admire your strength and love. You're my role model, my guiding light. I'm so grateful for the sacrifices you've made for me and for the love you've always given me.

I'll be here for you every step of the way, holding your hand, listening to you, and supporting you. I love you more than words can express.

WITH ALL MY LOVE

Get Involved

Breast Cancer Awareness

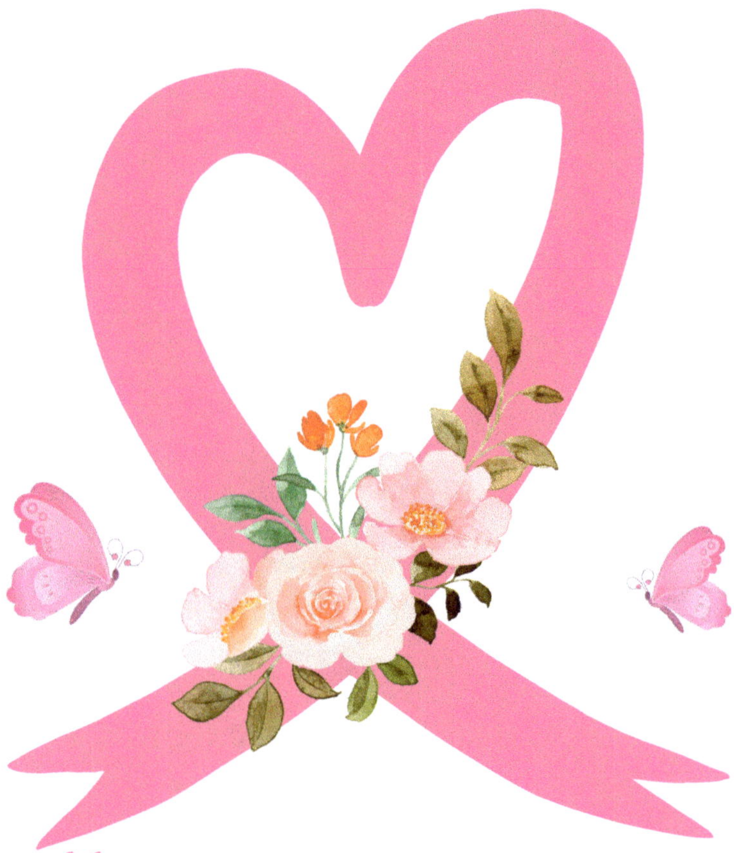

Join local breast cancer awareness walks or fundraisers to support research and survivors.

Share your story or support a loved one impacted by breast cancer.

Wear pink to support the fight against breast cancer.

Early detection saves lives!

BREAST CANCER MEDICAL GLOSSARY

Arm yourself with knowledge: A breast cancer glossary to help you understand your diagnosis, treatment options, and journey ahead.

	Medical term	Medical Meaning
R	Reconstruction	Surgery to rebuild the breast after mastectomy.
O	Oncologist	A doctor specializing in cancer treatment.
M	Mastectomy	Surgery to remove one or both breast
M	Mammogram	An x-ray of the breast tissue to detect abnormalities.
L	Lumpectomy	Surgery to remove the tumor and some surrounding tissue.

	Medical Term	Medical Meaning
PR	Pathology Report	Detailed report on tissue examination and diagnosis
B	Benign	Non-cancerous growths or tumors
T	Tumor	Abnormal growth of tissue (benign or cancerous)
HT	Hormone Therapy	Treatment to block hormones fueling cancer growth.
CT	Clinical Trial	Research study testing new treatments or approaches

May this breast cancer medical glossary empower readers with knowledge. May it help with improving communication with healthcare providers. May it reduce anxiety and uncertainty. I hope it supports education and understanding. Including a medical glossary in this booklet will help make medical information more accessible.

I am sending a heartfelt thank you for spending time with this booklet, and for being part of the effort to bring awareness,
knowledge, and hope for breast cancer.

Every small step we take together helps to spread understanding, encourage support, and uplift those who need it most. Awareness
does not stop here.

Please share this booklet with friends, family, and your community. Together, we can spark conversations, provide comfort, and remind others
that no one walks this journey alone. If you found
encouragement in these activities, I invite you
to explore more of my books, each designed to inspire
reflection, healing, and growth.

With Gratitude and Hope,
Delatria Sam
Author, Loved One

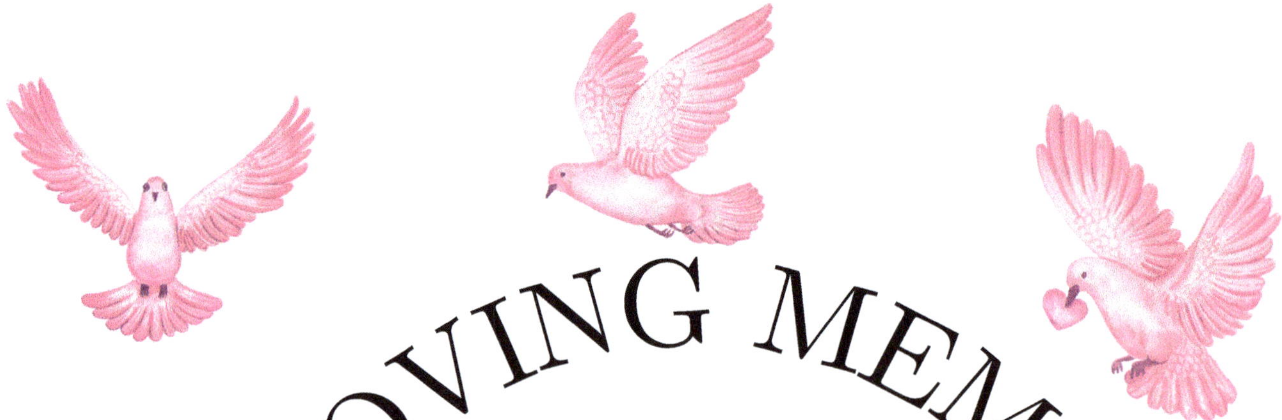

IN LOVING MEMORY

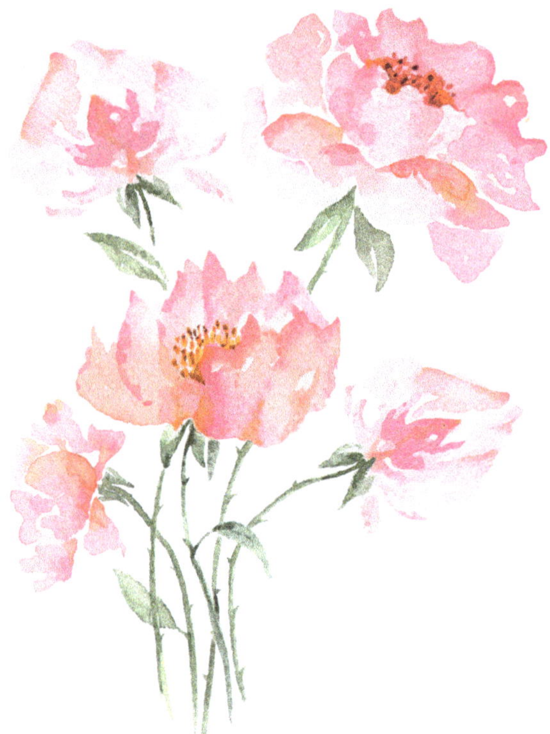

Honoring the strength, courage, and love of those who have fought bravely against breast cancer. May their legacy inspire us to continue the fight for a world without breast cancer.

Together, we support and strive for a future where breast cancer no longer takes lives.

www.ingramcontent.com/pod-product-compliance
Lightning Source LLC
LaVergne TN
LVHW070858210926
848482LV00016B/967

* 9 7 9 8 3 3 0 3 2 0 4 6 2 *